Sameh Sayhi
Sameh Mezri

Adverse effects of corticosteroid therapy in lupus

Sameh Sayhi
Sameh Mezri

Adverse effects of corticosteroid therapy in lupus

Systemic erythematosus

ScienciaScripts

Cover image: www.ingimage.com

This book is a translation from the original published under ISBN 978-620-6-71604-4.

Publisher:
Sciencia Scripts
is a trademark of
Dodo Books Indian Ocean Ltd. and OmniScriptum S.R.L publishing group

120 High Road, East Finchley, London, N2 9ED, United Kingdom
Str. Armeneasca 28/1, office 1, Chisinau MD-2012, Republic of Moldova, Europe
Managing Directors: Ieva Konstantinova, Victoria Ursu
info@omniscriptum.com

Printed at: see last page
ISBN: 978-620-8-55532-0

Contents

1 INTRODUCTION

The anti-inflammatory properties of corticoids have a long history in medical practice. In fact, these synthetic hormones have continued to work wonders in a number of medical and surgical specialities thanks to their powerful anti-inflammatory and immunosuppressive actions, to the point where general corticosteroid therapy is now one of the most widespread therapies in the world. [1]

In a department of internal medicine, corticosteroids are the first-line therapy and the key element in the management of most chronic inflammatory diseases, including systemic lupus erythematosus (SLE). SLE is a non-organ-specific autoimmune disease that can be life-threatening. Corticosteroid therapy is a fundamental therapeutic tool in the treatment of relapses of SLE.

Despite the many beneficial effects of these molecules, their use is limited as far as possible because of their side-effects. Corticosteroid therapy can give rise to potentially serious metabolic, infectious and osteoarticular complications. However, the adverse effects of corticosteroids are often avoidable or can be minimised.

This makes the choice of corticosteroid therapy a delicate one, based on an acceptable balance between sufficient anti-inflammatory activity and tolerable side effects. [3]

The objectives of our study are :

- Be aware of the various adverse effects inherent in corticosteroid therapy.
- Determine the role of the nurse in the management of a patient on corticosteroid therapy.

2 MATERIALS AND METHODS

I. **Scope of the study :**

Our study was conducted in the internal medicine department of the Hôpital Militaire Principal de Tunis (HMPIT).

II. **Type and period of study :**

1. Type of study :

This was a retrospective descriptive study.

2. Study period :

The study is being carried out over a two-month period from February to March 2016.

III. **Patients :**

1. Inclusion criteria :

All lupus patients who were hospitalised and treated with systemic corticosteroids, and who were hospitalised between June 2012 and December 2015.

2. Exclusion criteria :

Lupus patients not taking systemic corticosteroids.

IV. **Methods :**

1. Data collection :

- To collect the data, we used a pre-established form containing all the variables from the hospital records.
- Data were collected from 75 patients of different ages and genders.
- This study sheet includes epidemiological (age, gender), clinical (clinical form of SLE), therapeutic (corticosteroid treatment: molecule, dose, duration, method of administration) and evolutionary data for each patient and the list of adverse effects of this treatment.

2. Data analysis :

We carried out an analytical study and summarised the results for these patients. The data was entered and analysed using Excel 2007 and word processing using Word 2007.

3 RESULTS

I. EPIDEMIOLOGICAL DATA :

Of the 90 lupus patients admitted to hospital, 75 were being treated with systemic corticosteroids.

I.1.Age :

The mean age of our patients at the time of the study was 41.16 years, with extremes ranging from 16 to 84 years.

Forty-four percent of the lupus population studied fell into the 30-45 age bracket.

Figure 1 shows the distribution of patients by age:

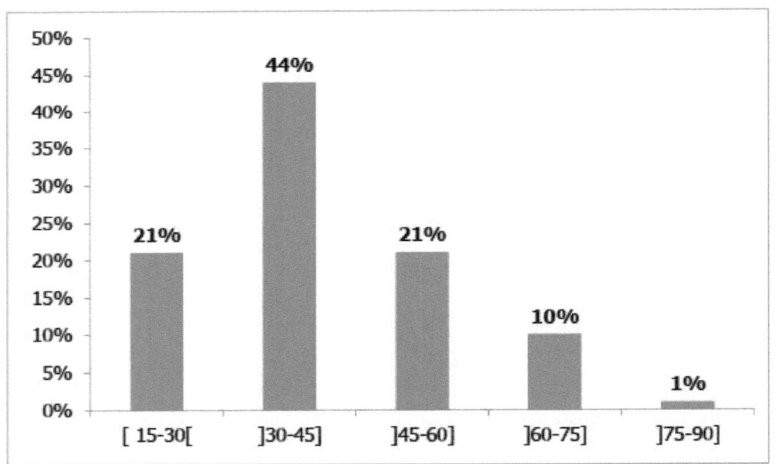

Figurei: Distribution of patients by age at the time of the study.

I.2.Genre :

Our series comprised 57 women and 18 men. The sex ratio F/M was 3.16.

Figure 2 shows the distribution of patients by gender.

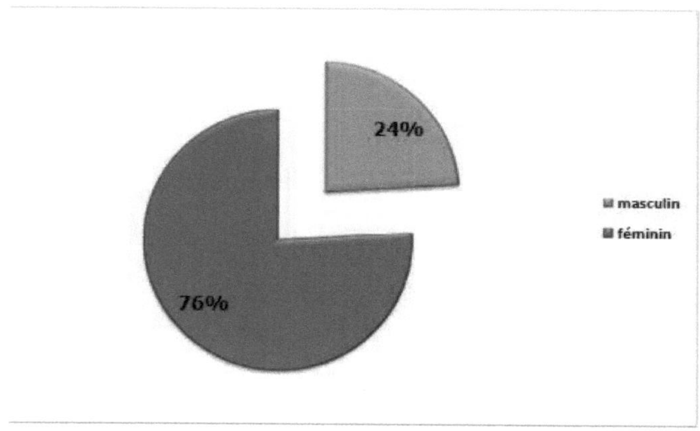

Figure 2: Breakdown of patients by gender.

II. CLINICAL DATA :

Clinical form of SLE :

- Mucocutaneous involvement was prescribed in 66 patients, i.e. **80%**, most of whom developed vespertilial erythema.
- Rheumatological complaints were reported in 71 patients (**95%)**, of whom 41 had arthralgia, 24 had arthritis and the remaining 6 had myalgia.
- Neurological damage was prescribed in 23 patients (**31%**), whose various symptoms were of central nervous system damage such as: convulsive seizures, gait disturbance, consciousness disturbance, mental confusion, vertigo, headache, temporo-spatial disorientation ....
- Digestive problems were present in 15 patients (**20%)**, in the form of abdominal pain, diarrhoea, haemorrhagic gastropathy and pancreatitis.

Cardiac intervention was prescribed in 29 patients (**37%),** 14 of whom had presented with pericarditis and functional signs such as chest pain and dyspnoea on exertion. The other patients had presented with other manifestations such as:

valvulopathy with mitral insufficiency, myocarditis....

- Pulmonary involvement was prescribed in 21 patients (**28%),** with cases of pleurisy and pleural effusion.

- Renal impairment was prescribed in 50 patients (**67%),** with manifestations of class I and IV lupus nephropathy and different classes of glomerulonephritis.

-Figure 3 shows the different clinical manifestations.

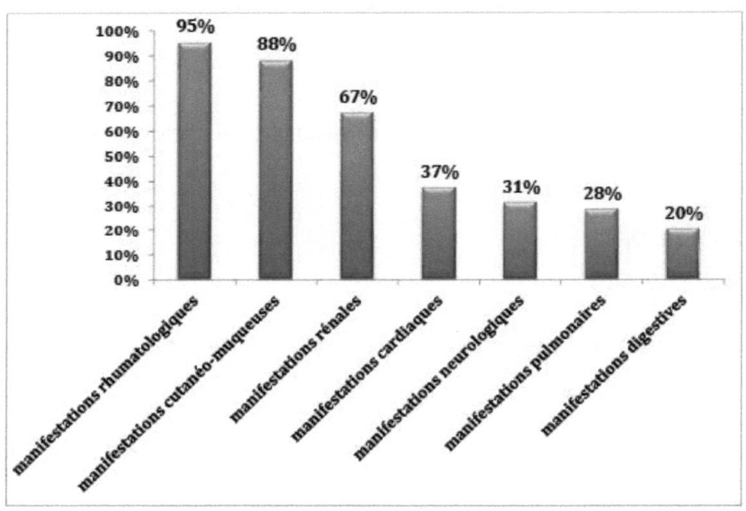

Figure 3: Distribution of patients according to clinical form.

CORTI^DES TREATMENT :

III.1. I.Molecules :

-Methylprednisolone (Solumedrol) was administered intravenously in 34 patients at the start of treatment in the form of a bolus, followed by prednisone (1mg/kg/day). Fifty-five per cent of patients received corticosteroid treatment in tablet form. Prednisone (cortancyl) and prednisolone (solupred) were prescribed orally in 35 and 21 patients respectively.

III.2. 2 The dose :

- A dose of lmg/kg/d of prednisone was prescribed in 41 cases **(55%)**, indicated for joint manifestations.
- A dose of 0.5mg/Kg/d was prescribed for 12 patients whose indication was serositis (pleurisy, pericarditis).
- A dose of 10-20mg/Kg/d was prescribed in 22 patients with non-erosive polyarthritis.

Table 1 shows corticosteroid treatment as a function of dose.

Dose	**10-20mg/kg**	**1mg/kg**	**0.5mg/kg**
Workforce	22	41	12
Percentage	***29%***	***55%***	***16%***

Table 1: Corticosteroid treatment according to dose.

III.3. 3. duration :

Seventy of lupus patients received systemic corticosteroid therapy for a period of one month or more for various clinical conditions: cardiac, neurological, renal, etc.

Table 2 shows corticosteroid treatment as a function duration.

Duration	**short: less than one month**	**long: greater than or equal to one month**
Workforce	5	70
Percentage	***7%***	***93%***

Table 2: Corticosteroid treatment according to duration.

For the five lupus patients who received short-term corticosteroids, the indication was disabling polyarthralgia or non-erosive polyarthritis.

IV. THE UNDESIRABLE EFFECTS OF CORTICTHERAPY :

Eighty-seven **percent (87%)** of patients treated with corticosteroids had experienced adverse reactions to the treatment.

Figure 4 shows the various side effects of corticosteroid therapy:

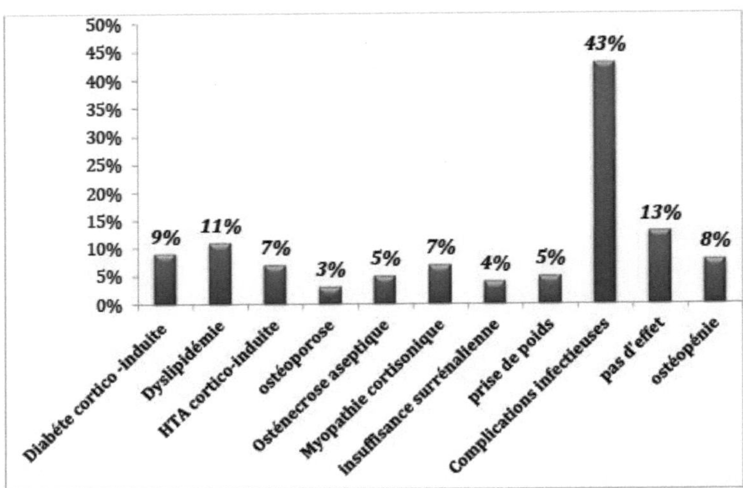

Figure 4: Side effects of corticosteroid therapy.

IV.1. Infectious complications :

Thirty-two patients presented with infectious complications, representing **43%** of complications.

- Twenty-two patients had a bacterial infection with :

J Eighteen cases of urinary tract infection, i.e. **24%** of our patients: 14 with E. coli, 4 with klebsiella

J Two cases of pneumoniaone of which developed severe sepsis requiring transfer to intensive care.

J Two cases of tuberculosis were reported, one of which was multifocal.

- Seven were viral infections, 3 of which were cases of herpes zoster.
- Three, mycotic infections, representing **4%** of patients.

Corticosteroid therapy: side effects

These patients require systemic antibiotic therapy, but the outcome is not always favourable: some patients have worsening renal function, leading to renal failure and dialysis, while others progress to death.

Figure 5 shows the distribution of infections according to the nature of the pathogen:

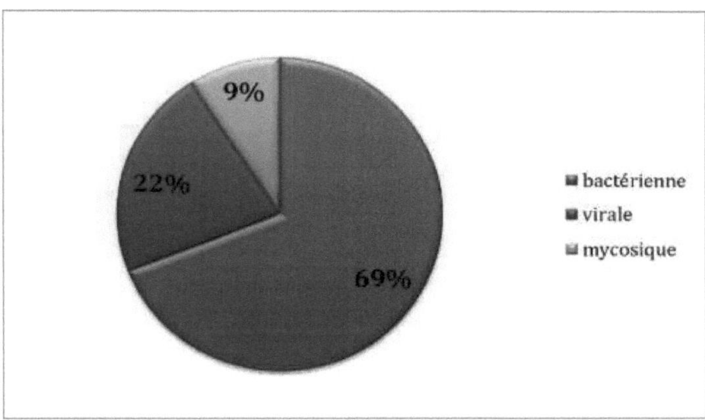

Figure 5: Distribution infections according to the nature of the pathogen.

IV.2 Bone complications :

-Bone complications were observed in 13 cases (**16%** of patients).

❖ Bone densitometry (BMD), performed in 12 patients, showed :

- Osteoporosis of the spine and lumbar vertebrae, uncomplicated by fracture, was present in 2 patients (**3%** of cases).
- Osteopenia was present in 6 patients (**8%)**.
- Aseptic osteonecrosis of the femoral head was noted in 4 lupus patients (3 women and 1 man), i.e. **5%** of the population studied. These patients complained of hip or thigh pain with limping on walking.

Figure 6 shows the bone complications of corticosteroid therapy:

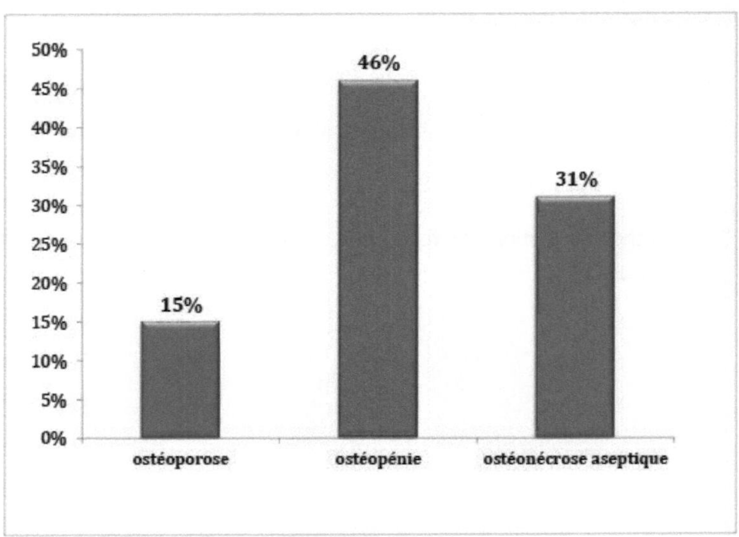

Figure 6: Bone complications of corticosteroid therapy.

One patient required a hip replacement.

Corticosteroid therapy: side effects

IV.3 Metabolic complications :

Twenty patients had one or more metabolic complications (cortico-induced diabetes, cortico-induced hypertension, dyslipidemia), i.e. **26%** of all patients:

IV.3.1. Cortico-induced diabetes :

Seven patients (five women and two men) had presented with cortico-induced diabetes or glucose intolerance, i.e. **9%** of the cases studied.

The average time to onset of this metabolic complication was 4 months.

Four patients with an HbA1c greater than 9% who had received antidiabetic treatment.

Only one patient presented with decompensation of diabetes.

IV.3.2 Cortico-induced hypertension :

Five patients developed hypertension, i.e. **7%** of the cases studied, with two patients having decompensated a pre-existing hypertension requiring the reinforcement of antihypertensive treatment.

IV.3.3 Dyslipidemia :

Eight cases of dyslipidaemia were confirmed (5 women, 3 men), representing **40%** of all metabolic complications.

The lipid profile showed an increase in total cholesterol and triglyceride levels with :

- Five cases of hypercholesterolaemia.
- Only one case of triglycerides.
- Two mixed cases.

Some patients were on statin therapy.

Figure 7 summarises the various metabolic complications of corticosteroid therapy:

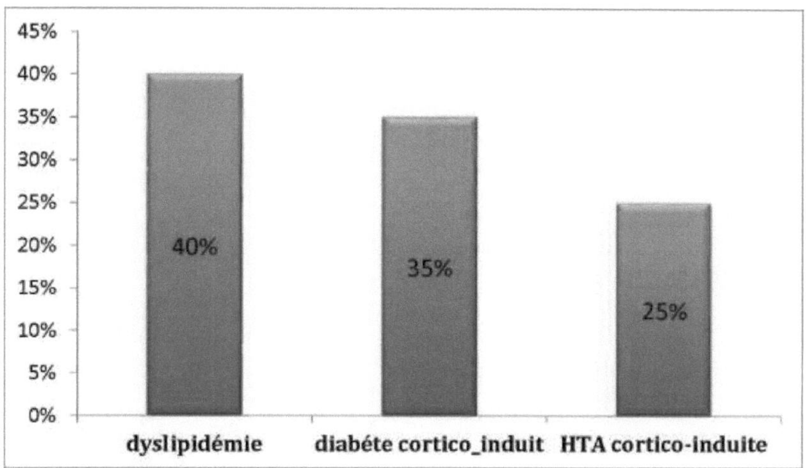

Figure 7: Metabolic complications of corticosteroid therapy.

IV.4. Cortisonic myopathies :

Myopathy was noted in 5 patients, i.e. **7%** of cases.

Muscle enzymes (CPK, LDH, AS AT...) increase in cortisone myopathy.

IV.5. Endocrine complications :

IV.5.1 Adrenal insufficiency:

Three patients had developed adrenal insufficiency, which was symptomatic when corticosteroid therapy was stopped. Two of these patients required hospitalisation.

IV.5.2 Cushing's syndrome:

Four patients presented with a cushingoid facies, i.e. 5% of the patients followed.

4 Discussion

1. *Corticoids :*

1. Definition of corticoids :

Corticoids are anti-inflammatory, pain-relieving and anti-redematous **drugs** used in a wide range of diseases. These molecules are synthesised from cortisol, a natural hormone produced by the **adrenal cortex**. [24]

2. Definition of corticosteroid therapy :

Corticotherapy is the administration of glucocorticoid substances for therapeutic purposes. [5]

3. Classification of corticoids :

A distinction must be made between natural glucocorticoids and synthetic glucocorticoids.

> ***Natural glucocorticoids :***

Natural glucocorticoids (cortisone or hydrocortisone) are used primarily in hormone replacement therapy for adrenal insufficiency.

Hydrocortisone hemisuccinate, on the other hand, has a very rapid effect and should therefore be reserved for emergencies.

> ***Synthetic glucocorticoids*** :

Synthetic glucocorticoids have an increased activity in order to improve their anti-inflammatory action and their mineralocorticoid effects are reduced (table3). They are used in other therapeutic indications (anti-inflammatory, immunosuppressive, antiallergic) and are defined as :

> Short-acting corticoids (prednisone, prednisolone, methylprednisolone), with 4 to 5 times the anti-inflammatory power of cortisol;

> Corticoids with intermediary effects (triamcinolone, paramethasone), with 5 to 10 times the anti-inflammatory power of cortisol;

> Long-acting corticoids (betamethasone, dexamethasone, cortivazol), with 25 to 30 times the anti-inflammatory power of cortisol (up to 60 times for cortivazol). [6]

	Anti-inflammatory activity	**Mineral-corticoid activity**	**Dose equivalence**	**Biological half-life (hours)**
Hydrocortisone	1	1	20 mg	8-12
Cortisone	0.8	1	25 mg	8-12
Prednisone and Prednisolone	4	0.8	5 mg	12-36
Methylprednisolone	5	0.5	4 mg	12-36
Triamcinolone	5	0	4 mg	12-36
Betamethasone	25	0	0.75 mg	36-54
Dexamethasone	25	0	0.75 mg	36-54
Cortivazol	60	0	0.3 mg	>60

Table 3: Glucocorticoid activity. [7]

4. Pharmacodynamic properties :

-Therapeutic properties :

- **Anti-inflammatory action**:

Corticosteroid therapy: side effects

The anti-inflammatory activity is exerted on the different phases of the inflammatory reaction, and is seen at low doses (0.1 mg/kg/day of prednisone equivalent). Corticosteroids reduce :

Production of pro-inflammatory cytokines ;

The synthesis of other inflammatory mediators and inhibit the action of adhesion molecules;

The differentiation and anti-infectious activity of macrophages.

- **Anti-allergic and immunosuppressive action**:

These two actions require higher doses than the anti-inflammatory action. Corticoids reduce the number of circulating T lymphocytes, as well as the production, proliferation and function of helper, suppressor and cytotoxic T lymphocytes.

- **Vasoconstrictor action**:

Corticoids have their own vasoconstrictive effect, independent of the previous effects, particularly on cutaneous vessels. They reduce capillary permeability. [6]

5. Pharmacokinetics

i- Absorption :

-The digestive absorption (in the initial part of the jejunum) of prednisone is rapid, approximately 80% by the oral route after a single dose. After absorption, prednisone is converted to the active metabolite prednisolone by 11ß-hydroxylation in the liver. However, prednisolone metasulfobenzoate (Solupred®) is less well absorbed than prednisone (Cortancyl®), which makes it less bioavailable. As a result, prednisone is preferred in the treatment of inflammatory diseases.

4- Protein binding :

In plasma, the majority of glucocorticoids circulate in bound form (**90%** for prednisone and prednisolone, **77%** for methylprednisolone) to two transport proteins: albumin, which has a high capacity but low affinity, and transcortin or "Cortisol Binding Globulin" (CBG), an alpha 2 globulin with a low capacity but high affinity.

4- Elimination

- Glucocorticoid molecules are lipophilic and must be metabolised into more water-soluble metabolites before they can be eliminated. Elimination is mainly via the kidneys. [24]

6. Indications for corticosteroids :

Corticosteroids have a wide range of indications:

J Systemic inflammatory diseases: (in their severe forms, with multiviceral involvement)

- Systemic lupus erythematosus (as in our series)
- rheumatoid arthritis
- Still's disease...

Vasculitis

Autoimmune bullous dermatoses (pemphigus, bullous pemphigoid)

Neurological disorders :

- multiple sclerosis
- spinal cord injuries
- myasthenia gravis.

o In our series, we were interested in the study of SLE because it represents an important indication for long-term corticosteroid therapy. The study by Chaachoui Fatma et al found that corticosteroids were indicated in 60% of lupus patients [9]. In our series, corticosteroid therapy was indicated in 80% of cases.

Corticosteroid therapy: side effects

7. Contraindications:

There is no absolute contraindication to brief corticosteroid therapy or corticosteroid therapy for vital purposes.

- Known allergy.
- Peptic ulcer disease.
- Uncontrolled infectious conditions.
- Uncontrolled psychotic states.
- Progressive viral diseases [8].

II. Epidemiology

❖ ***Age :***

-Most lupus patients who had received systemic corticosteroids were between 30 and 45 years of age, with an average age of 41.16 years. In the literature, a retrospective study, between January 2006 and June 2009 in the internal medicine department of CHU Mohamed VI, focused on patients who had received systemic corticosteroid therapy for at least three months and at doses >7.5mg prednisone equivalent, The average age was: 35.75 years (17--> 70ans). [1]

❖ ***Genre :***

-We found a predominance of women (**76%),** which could be explained by hormonal (restrogens) and genetic (x chromosome) factors. [10]. This result is similar to a study by the National Reference Centre for SLE, Professor Amoura's department of internal medicine at the Hôpital de la Pitié, Paris [10], which found a female predominance of **88.3%** compared with **11.7%.**

Corticosteroid therapy: side effects

III. ***Undesirable effects of corticosteroid therapy :***

1. Risk of infection :

- Infections are the consequence of reduced resistance to bacterial, viral, parasitic or fungal agents, induced by corticosteroids - evident from 20 mg per day of prednisone equivalent - and, possibly, immunosuppression linked to the underlying disease or associated therapies and morbid conditions. It may be the relapse of a latent, "locked-in" infection (tuberculosis, anguillosis, toxoplasmosis, herpes, shingles, etc.) or a superinfection, sometimes due to an opportunistic germ. Superinfections often have poor presenting symptoms, and should be suspected in the presence of any isolated persistent fever. As corticoids cause neutrophil hyperleukocytosis, this biological disturbance alone does not constitute an argument in favour of a septic process. [12]

-In our series, infectious complications were the most frequent complication with 32 cases, i.e. almost **43%** of complications. Their frequency in the literature varies between 26 and **78% [**13**]**. This frequency was comparable to a retrospective study carried out in the internal medicine department of Sfax (Tunisia) on 146 lupus patients hospitalised over an 11-year period from January 1996 to December 2006 [14].

-The causative infectious agent was identified in 111 cases **(76%**):

> Bacterial infections were the most common, occurring in 75 cases **(67.5%),** and in **68.75% of** our cases.

> Viral infections were observed in 12 cases **(10.8%)**.

> Other infections were parasitic in 15 cases **(13.5%)** and mycotic in 9 cases **(8%).**

○ So susceptibility to infection is increased by glucocorticoids.

Corticosteroid therapy: side effects

-I- Role of the nurse :

To prevent and detect these risks, the nurse should :

- administer prophylactic antibiotic therapy as prescribed by a doctor
- monitor temperature and any signs of infection (coughing, burning, urinary tract

infections, etc.)

- treat all wounds and infections
- observe rigorous hygiene
- make sure your vaccinations are up to date
- monitor their effectiveness = absence of pain and allergic reaction [15].
- A full work-up should be carried out for any fever not clearly linked to a lupus attack [12], including an infectious disease work-up (blood count, CRP, PCT, etc.).

2. Bone and muscle complications :

2.1- Cortisone-induced osteoporosis :

Cortisone-induced osteoporosis is the most common form of secondary osteoporosis and is one of the main complications of long-term cortisone therapy. However, an epidemiological study showed that only **14%** of patients taking long-term corticosteroid therapy were receiving preventive or curative treatment for cortisone-induced osteoporosis. There is a rapid increase in the risk of fracture in the first six months of any systemic corticosteroid treatment. The risk of osteoporosis decreases from the third month after stopping corticosteroid treatment. [16]

- Our study showed that 12 cases had bone complications confirmed by DMO, no case of osteoporotic fracture was reported, representing **16%** of the population.
- **I- Role of the nurse :**
- To prevent and detect these risks, the nurse had to :

o Monitor for the appearance of bone and joint pain

Corticosteroid therapy: side effects

o Calcaemia and calciuria on medical prescription

o Avoid activities where there is a risk of falling

o Calcium supplementation on medical prescription [15] o Ensuring a calcium-rich diet

2.2- Cortisonic myopathy :

-Cortisone myopathy was recognised as a side effect of corticosteroid therapy in 1955, shortly after this class of drugs was introduced into therapy. [21] Muscle weakness of varying severity is frequently observed in patients treated for several weeks with high doses of corticosteroids. Studies have shown that **15** to **40%** of patients treated with high doses of corticoids for several weeks suffer from this undesirable effect of treatment. However, this muscular damage is usually moderate and disabling in less than **5%** of patients. The frequency of tendon damage is unknown but appears to be rare, whereas in our series cortisone myopathy represents a minimal percentage of **7%.** [18]

-1- Role of the nurse :

-To prevent and detect these risks, the nurse should :

- Monitor the onset of walking difficulties
- Maintain coordination with the physiotherapist
- Ensure follow-up with complementary examinations
- Ensure a protein-rich diet

3. Metabolic complications :

-In our study, 20 metabolic complications were identified, i.e. **26%** of patients had one or other of these complications.

Corticosteroid therapy: side effects

3.1- Diabetes:

-All the effects of glucocorticoids on glucose metabolism contribute to hyperglycaemia. They increase hepatic glucose production, notably by increasing the availability of neoglucogenesis precursors and stimulating glucagon secretion. They also cause muscular insulin resistance by reducing peripheral glucose utilisation and oxidation. Finally, they have a direct toxic effect on beta cells. Glycaemic targets will depend on the context: age, underlying pathology, etc. It seems reasonable to set glycaemic targets of between 1.5 and 2.5 g/l in the elderly, lower: < 1.2 g/l fasting, < 1.6 g/l postprandial in the young. [17]

Some studies have estimated that 5-10% of patients treated with corticosteroids develop diabetes after more than a year of treatment. This is 1.5 to 2 times higher than the figure observed in a population of the same age not treated with cortisone. [18]

-1- Role of the nurse :

-To prevent and detect this diabetogenic risk, the nurse had to :

- Screen for signs of hypoglycaemia (palpitations, pallor, nausea, intense fatigue, sweating, tremors, vagal discomfort) and hyperglycaemia (hunger, intense thirst, polyuria, glycosuria)
- Monitor capillary glycaemia
- Follow a diabetic diet as prescribed by your doctor (avoid rapidly absorbed sugars, sweets and pastries).
- Administer an oral antidiabetic on prescription or implement insulin therapy [15].

3.2- Cortico-induced hypertension :

Prolonged systemic corticosteroid therapy may induce secondary hypertension or aggravate it if it is pre-existing.

- Arterial hypertension is diagnosed in **10** to **20%** of patients treated with corticosteroids, most often after several months of treatment. [18]
- In our study, hypertension appears to be induced in almost **7%** of patients.

Corticosteroid therapy: side effects

- A retrospective study carried out between January 2006 and June 2009 in the internal medicine department of the Mohamed VI University Hospital, Marrakech, showed that hypertension was noted in **6.94%** of cases, which appears to be equivalent to our study. [1]

- Role of the nurse :

-To prevent and detect this risk, the nurse should :

- Maintain a salt-free diet (avoid adding cooking salt, foods containing hidden salt, fizzy drinks) [15].
- Intervening in the event of a hypertensive peak
- Administer high blood pressure treatment as prescribed by a doctor

3.3- Hpidic blan disturbances :

- In our study, 8 cases had confirmed hyperlipidaemia, representing a percentage of **11%**.
- A prospective study carried out by L.FARDET's team aimed to describe changes in lipid levels under general corticosteroid therapy [1]. This study included 45 patients between June 2003 and May 2005, all of whom had received prolonged corticosteroid therapy lasting more than 3 months and high initial doses (mean: 54±17 mg/d) of prednisone, and who were not receiving any treatment that could have an influence on lipid levels. The results concluded that total cholesterol and triglyceride levels increased: from 1.79 g/l to 2.38 g/l and from 1.02 g/l to 1.16 g/l respectively between D0 and M3 of systematic corticosteroid therapy, and fell at the end of treatment.

A pre-treatment check-up was carried out (total cholesterol, HDL, LDL, triglycerides) and after three months of treatment. Forty-two patients had complete lipid analyses at three months, and 21 of them also had them at 9 to 12 months. [19]

Date	Day 1	At 3 months	Between 9 and 12 months
Prednisone dose (mg/day)	54+/-17	31+/-15	11+/-6
Cholesterol levels Average (in g/l)	1.79	2.38	2.10
HDL cholesterol	67% increase		
LDL cholesterol	17% increase		
Triglyceridemia (in g/l)	1.02	1.16	0.96

HDL=High density lipoproteins

LDL=Low density lipoproteins

Table 5: Study of lipid levels in patients taking corticosteroids. [19]

-1- Role of the nurse :

- To prevent and detect this risk, the nurse should:

○ Carry out a lipid profile (cholesterol, triglycerides) on the basis of a doctor's prescription, while complying with the dosage rules (12-hour fasting period) [15].

○ Ensure a hypolipidemic diet by reducing calories or treatment under medical prescription

4. Cortico-induced adrenal insufficiency:

First described in the 1950s, cortico-induced adrenal insufficiency is a classic side-effect of systemic corticosteroid therapy. It is currently even unanimously considered to be the leading cause of secondary adrenal insufficiency. [1]

-In fact, when corticoids are taken for long periods of time and ACTH and cortisol secretions have been put to rest, the adrenal glands may rest and often even atrophy.

The intensity of inhibition will depend on the compound, the dose, the duration of treatment and the time of administration. Insufficiency may be due either directly to the adrenal glands being put to rest, or {to the pituitary gland not resuming secretion of ACTH}.

Adrenal insufficiency may occur with long-term oral corticosteroid therapy, but fortunately it is rare (incidence between **0.015** and **0.1%**). [20]

○ In our series, 3 cases were confirmed, i.e. **4%** of the population. A prospective study of 56 patients (June 2011 to December 2012) receiving prolonged oral corticosteroid therapy with a mean initial prednisone dose of 50+/-22 mg/day. Adrenal insufficiency was observed in 36 cases (**64%**). Several studies have estimated the frequency of biological IS in patients receiving long-term corticosteroid therapy to be between **15** and **87%.** [20]

-I- Role of the nurse :

To prevent and detect these risks, the nurse should :

- Gradually reduce the final dosage of corticosteroid therapy on medical prescription
- Administer the treatment between 7 and 8 in the morning, as the hormone corresponds to the maximum function of the adrenal glands, thus limiting the side effects.
- Biological monitoring adrenal function on medical prescription (synacthen test) [15].
- Screen for symptoms of adrenal insufficiency (unusual fatigue, abdominal pain, weight loss, sometimes fever) [18].

5. Ocular complications :

-Local and general corticoids are a source of serious ophthalmological complications, requiring regular ophthalmological monitoring adapted to the patient's history.

5.1. Cortisonic cataract :

-Cortisonic cataracts, which are generally posterior subcapsular, occur during local and especially prolonged corticosteroid therapy (average delay 1 year). This cataract may be favoured by general pathologies (diabetes) or ocular pathologies Corticosteroid therapy: undesirable effects

(uveitis, Fuchs' iris heterochromia). It is generally bilateral and sometimes asymmetric. It may stabilise or worsen when corticosteroids are stopped, reducing visual acuity. Treatment is surgical. [23]

5.2. Cortisonic glaucoma :

Cortisone-induced glaucoma is linked to an increase in ocular pressure associated with a reduction in the resorption of aqueous humour. This complication is mainly associated with local corticosteroid therapy, but can sometimes occur during high-dose systemic corticosteroid therapy. [23]

-I- Role of the nurse :

-To prevent and detect these risks, the nurse should :

- Question patients if there are any ocular signs
- Ensure ophthalmological follow-up

6. Digestive complications :

- Corticosteroids may induce certain digestive symptoms such as stomach pain/cramps or acid regurgitation. These symptoms are benign and can be easily treated by the doctor. The risk of more serious complications (stomach ulcer, inflammation of the pancreas, infection of the colon) is much lower. Around **10%** of patients complain of stomach pains at the start of treatment. The risk corticosteroid-induced stomach ulcers and pancreatitis is extremely low. On the other hand, corticosteroids may aggravate a pre-existing stomach ulcer. [18]

-I- Role of the nurse :

-To prevent and detect these risks, the nurse should :

- Monitor for the appearance of gastric pain such as burning or cramping.
- If prescribed by a doctor, administer a gastric dressing (2 hours before taking the corticosteroid so as not to interfere with absorption) or an antiulcer drug.
- Monitor post-gastric efficacy with antiulcer drugs away from meals, as food acts as a buffer and calms gastralgia.
- Avoid irritants (tobacco) + acidic foods (salad dressing, lemon, spices, etc.) No self-medication with ulcerogenic DTCs (NSAIDs, salicylic acid)
- Detect digestive haemorrhage (black blood in the stools). [15]

7. Psychiatric disorders :

-Mood changes induced by corticosteroids are usually minor (e.g. insomnia, anxiety or irritability, moderate memory problems, difficulty concentrating), but in rare cases may be more severe (e.g. depression, delusions, marked euphoria).

-Minor symptoms are common. For example, **40-50%** of patients report insomnia, irritability or anxiety. Severe neuropsychological disorders are much rarer, and may affect **5-10%** of patients. It is imperative that these disorders prompt patients (and/or those around them) to seek prompt medical advice. [18]

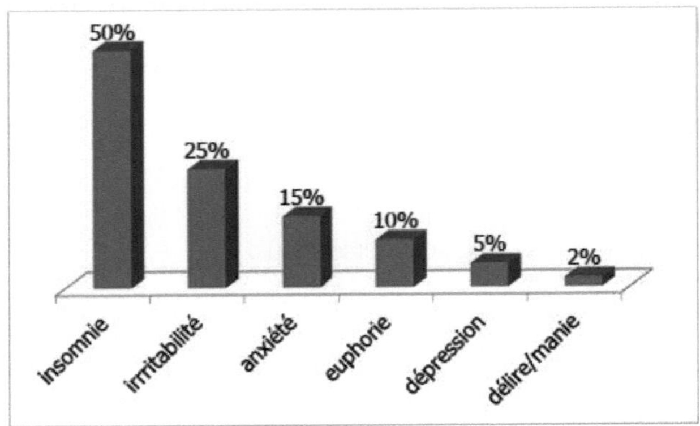

Figure 9: Mood changes. [18]

-I- Role of the nurse :

-To prevent and detect these risks, the nurse should :

- Monitor sleep quality
- Avoid all stimulants, particularly at the end of the day (coffee, tea, alcohol, tobacco).
- Monitor behaviour (mental confusion, hallucination) + risk of depression when treatment is stopped. [15]

7. Aesthetic complications :

-In our series, these side effects constituted a minimal percentage, i.e. **5%** of patients.

-Corticoids frequently induce weight . This weight is usually moderate, of the order of a few kilos. Corticosteroids also alter the physical appearance of the patient, with the appearance of a rounded face (the "moon face"), a hump at the nape of the neck (buffalo hump) or an increase in waist circumference. These anomalies are due to a redistribution of fat cells in the body (called lipodystrophy) and to water retention. It is estimated that after two to three months of treatment, 40 to 60% of patients will weight gain and/or a significant change in their physical appearance. [18]

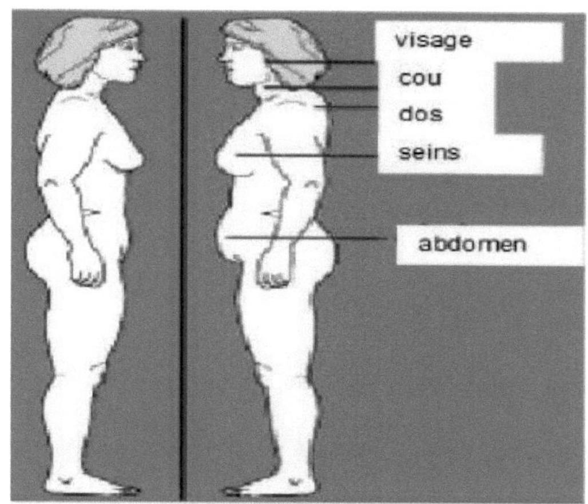

Before After

Figure 10: Weight gain. [18]

-Cushingoid facies is also known as "cervico-facial lipodystrophy" or "facio-truncular obesity", depending on the author, and four cases were reported in our study. A review of the literature (Table 7) confirms the high prevalence of this complication: ™ A study carried out in casa on patients treated with general corticosteroid therapy for various dermatological pathologies found cervico-facial lipodystrophy in all patients. [1]

studies made	Years	number of patients	Prevalence from case of lipodystrophy	median time to onset

Benchikhi & al	1999	72	100%	3 months
Flahault & al	2007	37	57%	3 months
Fardet & al	2007	88	63%	3 months
Study by Zineb BENNIS KANAR	2009	72	55.5%	3 months

Table 6: Comparison of the prevalences of cervicofacial lipodystrophy in the different studies mentioned above. [1]

-I- Role of the nurse :

-To prevent and detect these risks, the nurse should :

- Ensure a hypokalaemic diet on medical prescription (avoid animal and vegetable fats)
- Monitor weight
- Observe changes in body shape and the resulting psychological effects [15].

-Finally, we must not forget that the nurse must :

- Enabling people to express their feelings
- Providing psychological support (counselling)
- Enabling people to acquire the necessary knowledge about diets, daily activities and self-monitoring.
- Ensure an educational approach. [15]

Given the seriousness of the systemic diseases being treated, and the potential dangers of corticosteroid therapy, failure to monitor corticosteroid-treated patients would be serious medical negligence, and would be punishable by law. Monitoring patients is therefore an integral part of the basic rules of good corticosteroid therapy. The frequency of follow-up depends on the severity of the symptoms of the initial disease and on the patient's tolerance to corticosteroids. [1] Table 6 lists the various parameters to be monitored by questioning, clinical examination and additional tests.

Questioning	Clinic	Additional examinations
-appetite -treatment compliance -diet compliance -sleep disorders -psychological state -digestive signs -Osteoarticular signs	-blood pressure measurement -weight monitoring -temperature -growth chart (children++) ophthalmological examination with measurement of eye pressure -skin examination	-blood ionogram -fasting blood glucose -Protein levels -cholesterolemia -triglyceridemia -enumeration formula blood -osteodensitometry (start and 6 months)

Table 7:Signs of relapse of treated disease. [3]

5 Conclusion

The prescription of long-term corticosteroid therapy must be a carefully considered decision by the prescriber. He will need to assess the superiority of using a corticosteroid despite the risks of adverse effects, compared with the complications of the disease itself if treatment is not started. The search for the minimum effective dose will be the first line of defence against the risks of complications associated with corticosteroid therapy. [22]

Corticoids were undoubtedly one of the major advances in medical therapy of the last century. Thanks to them, many lives have been and continue to be saved every day for more than 60 years. Their rapid and spectacular effects on inflammation have revolutionised the prognosis of many dysimmune and inflammatory diseases that are often incapacitating. The other side of the coin is that this 'miracle treatment' has a long list of side-effects, which continue to grow with time.

The aim of this study, which focused on the harmful effects of corticoids, was to gain a better understanding of them so that we can deal with them more effectively.

It revealed that, although apparently well known, many of these adverse effects are far from being well understood in epidemiological and pathophysiological terms, let alone in terms of therapeutic management and preventive strategy, and that consensus recommendations are often sorely lacking.

Finally, and to conclude on a hopeful note, we would like to announce that in-depth research into the intracellular mechanisms of action of corticoids and their metabolism has enabled us to develop molecules that are just as powerful as our current corticoids, but without their side effects. These molecules are currently still at the pre-clinical stage. But who knows?

They will probably be tomorrow's revolution. [1]

6 Appendices

Connectivity study sheet

IDENTIFICATION :

Last name First name

Sex : M o

Ageyears old.

PERSONAL ANTECEDENTS :

Surgical :

SKIN AND MUCOUS MEMBRANES :

Purpura photosensitivity lupus discoid Raynaud's Mouth ulceration

Others :

Biopsy :

RHEUMATOLOGICAL MANIFESTATIONS :

Arthralgia : Headquarters

:....

Headquarters

Arthritis :

:....

Myalgias : Myositis :

KIDNEY EVENTS :

HTA Haematuria Proteinuria Redematous syndrome Anuria

Creatinine

PBR :

IRT :

Hemodialysis :

Digestive disorders :

Abdominal pain :

Diarrhoea :

Digestive perforation :

Ileocolitis :

Others :

Fibroscopy :

Colonoscopy :

Biopsy :

Cardiac manifestations :

Functional signs :

Cardiac auscultation :

ECG :

Chest X-ray :

ECHO CdUR :

Pericarditis Endocarditis Myocarditis PAH

OTHER :

PULMONARY MANIFESTATIONS :

Functional signs :

Review:

Rx thorax :

Chest scan :

Bronchial fibrosis :

Others :

NEUROLOGICAL MANIFESTATIONS :

Peripheral neuropathy :

EMG :

CNS involvement :

Cerebral CT :

Brain MRI :

TREATMENT :

CORTICOIDS :

Bolus :

Initial doses :

Duration :

ADVERSE DRUG REACTIONS :

EVOLUTION :

Improvement :

Worsening :

Stabilisation :

Fall :

Sequel :

Death : Cause:

7 References

[1] Zineb BENNIS KANAR. Complications of corticosteroid therapy Prolonged systemic treatment in internal medicine. Thesis N°69. MARRAKECH, CADI AYYAD UNIVERSITY 2010.

[2] Clémence HERBIN. METHODOLOGICAL PROBLEMS IN THE CLINICAL DEVELOPMENT OF AN IMMUNOMODULATOR IN LUPUS, A propos dune nouvelle molécule Atacicept dans la néphropathie lupique. PhD thesis. UNIVERSITE HENRI POINCARE - NANCY 1 2010.

[3] R. BERRADY, W. BONO. Service de Médecine Interne, CHU Hassan II, FES, MAROC.COMMENT JE PREVIENS LES EFFETS SECONDAIRES D'UNE CORTICOTHERAPIE BERRADY et COLL ANNALES DE MEDECINE ET DE THERAPEUTIQUE AMETHER. janvier 2010 ; Volume 2, N° 1 : 81 - 84

[4] KENTH D. BRANDT "Arthrose" Principe de médecine interne 15th edition Médecine science Flammarion Paris 1987-1994

[5] MAURICE RAPIN "Le grand dictionnaire Encyclopédique Médical" Tome 1, AH1986, Médecine et sciences Flammarion Paris France

[6] : www.scienceDirect.com

[7] Pharmacology Level DCEM1.2006 - 2007.Pharmacology Department Pr. Philippe Lechat. Updated: 18 October 2006. Chapter 14 - Corticosteroids.

[8] : www.soins-infirmiers.com. UPDATED:26/11/2008

[9]: Chaachoui Fatma. Monitoring a patient on corticosteroid therapy in an internal medicine department. End of study work 2013

[10] Laurent ARNAUD. Epidemiology of systemic lupus. Centre national de référence du lupus systémique Service de médecine interne 2 (Pr Amoura) Groupe hospitalier Pitié-Salpêtrière, Paris

[11] Rheumatology Department, Professor Olivier MEYER, DCEM2 course. Systemic lupus erythematosus: Diagnosis, evolution, principles of treatment. Module 8 Immunology Inflammation DCEM2 Internat n° 117

[12] Item 174 : Prescription and monitoring of steroidal and non-steroidal anti-inflammatory drugs. COFER, Collège Français des Enseignants en Rhumatologie. Document creation date 2010-2011.

[13] Mouna El Fane1, Meryem Essebani1, Wassila Bouissar2, Latifa Badaoui1, Ahd Oulad Lahsen1, Mustapha Sodqi1, Latifa Marih1, Abdelfettah Chakib1, Kamal Marhoum El Filali1. Infectious complications in systemic lupus erythematosus. Revue Marocaine de Rhumatologie 2015; 32: 39

[14] M. Michel *, B. Godeau. Infectious complications of systemic diseases. Department of Internal Medicine, CHU Henri-Mondor Hospital, 51, avenue du Maréchal-de-Lattre-de-Tassigny, 94010 Créteil cedex, France. Réanimation 14 (2005) 621-628

[15] :http://www.infirmiers.com/pdf/SI-personne-sous-corticoides.pdf

[16] MEDICATION TREATMENT OF CORTISONE-INDUCED OSTEOPOROSIS. Recommandation de Bonne Pratique. AGENCE FRANÇAISE DE SECURITE SANITAIRE DES PRODUITS DE SANTE EDITION DE

FEBRUARY 2003

[17] Diabetes and corticoids. Dr Florence LABROUSSE-LHERMINE Service de Diabétologie-Maladies Métaboliques et Nutrition CHU Rangueil.

[18] : http://www.cortisone-info.fr

[19] FARDET L., TIEV K.P., KETTANEH A., TOLEDANO C., CABANE J. "Corticothérapie systémique et perturbations du bilan lipidique: étude prospective ayant inclus 45 patients". La Revue de Médecine Interne. December 2006. Vol. 27, n°S3, p.S325.

[20] : http://scolarite.fmp-usmba.ac.ma/cdim/mediatheque/memoires/e_memoires/2-13.pdf

[21] T. Perez Pneumology and Immuno-Allergology Department, Hôpital Calmette, CHRU de Lille, 59037 Lille Cedex. Peripheral muscle and corticotherapy. Revue des Maladies Respiratoires vol 18, N° SUP 2 - May 2001pp. 234

[22] THESIS FOR THE STATE DIPLOMA OF DOCTOR OF PHARMACY. Presented and publicly defended on 21 November 2011 by Emilie BALDOMIR

[23] Bertrand Wechsler, Olivier Chosidow. Corticoids and corticosteroid therapy. John Libbey eurotext, 1997, Paris.

[24] http://www.docteurclic.com/traitement/corticoides.aspx

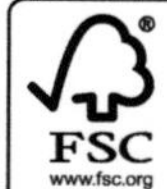
MIX
Papier aus verantwortungsvollen Quellen
Paper from responsible sources
FSC® C105338

Printed by Books on Demand GmbH, Norderstedt / Germany